Straight -To-The-Point

Alzheimer's

Management Guide Made Handy

By **CYNTHIA LEONARD**

TABLE OF CONTENTS

WHAT IS ALZHEIMER'S?

Alzheimer's disease is a progressive neurological condition that mostly affects elderly persons, however younger people may also have it. It is the most frequent cause of dementia, a collection of brain illnesses that cause memory loss and cognitive decline severe enough to impair day-to-day functioning.

Although the precise origin of Alzheimer's disease is unknown, a mix of lifestyle, environmental and genetic factors are thought to be involved. The aberrant buildup of tau tangles and beta-amyloid plaques in the brain, which impair nerve cell communication and ultimately cause their death, are two of the characteristic hallmarks of Alzheimer's disease.

Alzheimer's disease symptoms usually start off mildly—such as disorientation and memory loss—and become worse with time. Additional typical symptoms include trouble speaking, poor judgement, confusion, mood or behaviour swings and ultimately the inability to carry out everyday duties that are fundamental in nature.

Since there is currently no known cure for Alzheimer's, present therapies mainly aim to manage the disease's symptoms and delay its course. In an effort to better manage and eventually avoid this debilitating disorder, research into possible therapies and preventative strategies is still ongoing.

Causes and Risk Factors

A complicated disorder, Alzheimer's disease is brought on by a confluence of lifestyle, environmental and hereditary variables. Although the precise aetiology of Alzheimer's disease is still unknown, scientists have found a number of potential risk factors for the condition:

Genetic Elements:

Family history: Your risk is increased if you have a close relative, such a parent or brother, who has Alzheimer's.

Genetic mutations: The APOE-e4 gene is one gene that raises the risk of Alzheimer's disease. Nevertheless, the presence of these genes does not ensure that you will experience the illness.

Age: The biggest risk factor for Alzheimer's disease is becoming older. Growing older raises the chance of getting the illness, particularly beyond the age of 65.

Changes in the Brain: The buildup of aberrant proteins, such as tau tangles and beta-amyloid plaques, in the brain is a hallmark of Alzheimer's disease. These proteins cause a breakdown in nerve cell communication, which eventually results in tissue loss and cell death.

Environmental Elements: Alzheimer's disease risk may be raised by environmental variables such as exposure to pollutants, poisons or certain substances. Nevertheless, further investigation is required to comprehend the particular environmental elements at play.

Factors related to lifestyle:

Poor cardiovascular health: Alzheimer's disease risk has been associated with conditions that impact the heart and blood arteries, including high blood pressure, high cholesterol, diabetes and obesity.

Absence of Physical Activity: Alzheimer's disease risk may rise with a sedentary lifestyle.

Unhealthy Diet: Alzheimer's disease may develop as a result of a diet heavy in processed foods, refined carbohydrates and saturated fats.

Smoking: There is a link between smoking cigarettes and a higher risk of Alzheimer's disease.

Limited Cognitive Stimulation and Social Engagement: Reading, puzzles and social contact are good ways to keep the brain busy and lower the risk of cognitive decline.

Head Injury: A history of head trauma has been associated with a higher chance of acquiring Alzheimer's disease at a later age, especially if the damage was severe or repetitive.

While having these characteristics may raise one's chance of getting
Alzheimer's, having them does not ensure that one will get the illness.
Furthermore, it's possible that there are still unidentified elements
contributing to the onset of Alzheimer's disease.

Stages of the Disease

Typically, Alzheimer's disease develops in phases, each
with unique symptoms and difficulties. Note that every
person's experience with Alzheimer's disease is unique.

*The phases delineated underneath provide a comprehensive structure
for comprehending the customary advancement of the illness:*

Preclinical Stage: This phase may start years before any
symptoms become apparent. There are no overt
indications of cognitive loss during this period, while
aberrant proteins *(such as tau tangles and amyloid plaques)* are
building up in the brain.

Mild Cognitive Impairment (MCI): During this phase,
people may begin to exhibit subtle cognitive function

abnormalities that are apparent to them as well as to close friends or family members. These modifications might consist of:

- Forgetfulness, particularly with regard to recent exchanges or occurrences.

- Having trouble saying things or finishing what you know.

- Difficulties with organisation or planning.

Alzheimer's disease that is mild: The symptoms of Alzheimer's become worse with time and start to interfere more and more with day-to-day activities. At this point, common symptoms include:

- Growing memory loss, which includes losing track of significant occasions or private information.

- Difficulty making decisions and addressing problems.

- Uncertainty about location or time.

- Difficulties doing multi-step jobs, including handling funds or cooking.

- Alterations in mood and demeanour, such as heightened worry, agitation or retreat.

Moderate Alzheimer's Disease: During this phase, people may need more help with everyday tasks and have a more noticeable cognitive impairment. Among the symptoms might be:

- Severe memory loss, which includes losing track of important life events or the names of close family members.

- Having trouble identifying well-known faces or items.

- Difficulty doing everyday tasks like dressing or taking a shower.

- Wandering or becoming disoriented, even in familiar
  places.

- Alterations in behaviour, including anger, violence
  or hallucinations.

Alzheimer's Disease Severe: Significant cognitive
deterioration and the requirement for intensive assistance
and care are the hallmarks of this last stage. People in this
time might encounter:

- Total reliance on other people for everyday needs.

- Loss of verbal communication skills.

- Being incontinent.

- Trouble swallowing.

- Susceptibility to infections and other health
  problems is increased.

While these phases provide a broad picture of how Alzheimer's disease develops, not everyone will go through each stage precisely as outlined and the pace of advancement might differ greatly across people.

Diagnosis and Assessment

The process of diagnosing Alzheimer's disease entails a number of procedures, such as reviewing medical records, doing physical examinations, neurological examinations, and other testing to rule out other potential causes of symptoms.

An outline of the diagnostic and evaluation procedure is provided below:

Medical History Assessment: The doctor will inquire about the patient's symptoms, past medical conditions and family history of neurological illnesses such as Alzheimer's Disease.

Physical Examination: To evaluate general health and rule out any medical disorders that could be producing symptoms, a general physical examination will be performed.

Neurological Examination: To assess reflexes, muscular strength, coordination and sensory function, the physician will conduct a neurological examination. Also, they will evaluate cognitive abilities such as problem-solving, language, memory and attention.

Cognitive Testing: To evaluate memory, attention, language and other cognitive skills, cognitive tests like the Mini-Mental State Examination **(MMSE)** or the Montreal Cognitive Assessment **(MoCA)** may be used.

Laboratory Tests: To rule out further possible reasons of cognitive impairment, such as thyroid diseases, vitamin deficiencies or infections, blood tests may be performed.

Brain Imaging: Imaging studies, such as positron emission tomography **(PET)** or magnetic resonance imaging **(MRI)**, may be used to identify abnormalities in the brain linked to Alzheimer's disease, such as the presence of tau tangles and amyloid plaques.

Analysis of Cerebrospinal Fluid: A lumbar puncture, often known as a spinal tap, may be necessary in some circumstances to examine cerebrospinal fluid for Alzheimer's disease indicators, such tau and amyloid beta proteins.

Genetic Testing: To find genetic alterations linked to the illness, genetic testing may be advised in certain circumstances, particularly for those with a family history of early-onset Alzheimer's disease.

Functional Assessment: Information on the person's everyday functioning and any observable behavioural or personality changes may be requested from carers.

Follow-up and Monitoring: In order to follow the development of symptoms and modify treatment plans appropriately, it will be required to conduct continuing monitoring and evaluation if Alzheimer's disease is identified.

No one test can accurately detect Alzheimer's disease at this time. To rule out other possible causes of symptoms, diagnosis is often relied on a combination of clinical assessment, cognitive testing and other diagnostic procedures.

For those with Alzheimer's disease, an early diagnosis enables prompt intervention and therapy, which may help control symptoms and enhance quality of life.

RECOGNIZING SYMPTOMS AND TREATMENT

Diagnostic Tests and Evaluations

The following are a few typical diagnostic procedures and assessments used to identify Alzheimer's disease:

Medical history assessment includes learning about the patient's symptoms, past medical conditions and any family members who have had dementia or Alzheimer's disease. An extensive medical history may provide important information on the beginning and course of cognitive impairment.

Physical Examination: A comprehensive physical examination may assist determine general health and rule out other possible reasons of cognitive impairment. Reflexes, coordination and sensory function may all be assessed using neurological exams.

Cognitive Assessment: Memory, language, attention and executive function are just a few of the areas that are assessed by cognitive testing. Commonly used screening instruments for cognitive impairment include the Mini-Mental State Examination **(MMSE)** and the Montreal Cognitive Assessment **(MoCA).**

Neuropsychological Testing: Neuropsychological evaluations provide a more thorough analysis of cognitive abilities and may assist in differentiating between dementia kinds. These exams provide a detailed assessment of executive function, memory, language and visuospatial abilities.

Brain imaging: Studies using magnetic resonance imaging **(MRI)** and computed tomography **(CT)** scans may be used to see the structural alterations in the brain linked to Alzheimer's disease, including amyloid plaques and neurofibrillary tangles, brain shrinkage and other abnormalities.

By identifying aberrant protein deposits in the brain, amyloid or tau tracers used in Positron Emission Tomography **(PET)** scans may also help with the diagnosis.

Analysis of Cerebrospinal Fluid (CSF): A lumbar puncture may provide cerebrospinal fluid, which can be used to discover biomarkers suggestive of Alzheimer's disease. Aβ and tau protein levels in CSF are examples of biomarkers that may be used to demonstrate the existence of Alzheimer's disease pathology.

Genetic Testing: When there is a family history of early-onset Alzheimer's disease or other genetic risk factors, genetic testing could be advised. A genetic test for mutations in genes including **APP**, **PSEN1** and **PSEN2** may assist in determining who is more likely to have the illness.

Blood Tests: In order to rule out further possible reasons of cognitive impairment, such as infections, vitamin deficiencies or thyroid problems, blood tests may be carried out.

Functional Assessment: Assessing instrumental activities of daily living **(IADLs)** and activities of daily living **(ADLs)** may provide light on how cognitive decline affects a person's capacity to carry out daily chores on their own.

Psychiatric Evaluation: A mental health assessment is necessary to screen for mood disorders like anxiety or depression, which may exacerbate cognitive symptoms of Alzheimer's disease and coexist with the condition.

Importance of Early Detection

It is essential to identify Alzheimer's disease early for a number of reasons:

Treatment Planning: Early Alzheimer disease detection enables the start of suitable medical treatments and treatment regimens. Alzheimer's disease now has no known cure, although certain drugs and treatments may help control symptoms and halt the illness's development.

Early detection enables patients and their families to consider these choices and decide on the best course of treatment.

Optimising Quality of Life: People with Alzheimer's disease may better access resources and support services that can improve their quality of life when the condition is detected early. Programmes for cognitive stimulation, carer support groups and help with everyday tasks are a few examples of this. Individuals may sustain their independence and participate in worthwhile activities for extended periods of time by initiating these therapies early.

Putting Future Plans in Place: Alzheimer's disease is a degenerative illness that becomes worse with time. Early diagnosis enables people with Alzheimer's to continue to engage in decision-making, giving them and their family time to make future plans. This might include setting up advance directives for healthcare choices, talking about long-term care alternatives and arranging financial preparations.

Clinical Trials and Research: Participation in clinical trials and research studies aimed at creating new therapies and expanding our knowledge of the illness is made easier by early identification. Researchers can track the development of Alzheimer's and evaluate the efficacy of possible treatments by identifying people who are in the early stages of the illness.

Individuals who take part in clinical trials might also get experimental therapies that they would not otherwise be able to.

Reducing Carer Burden: In order to assist carers deal with the difficulties of caring, early diagnosis makes resources and support services available to them. It offers a chance for carers to become knowledgeable about the illness, create networks of support and learn useful coping mechanisms. Early attention to carer requirements may lessen the strain of caring and improve results for the individual with Alzheimer's disease as well as the carer.

All things considered, early identification of Alzheimer's disease is important to improving patient outcomes, raising quality of life and increasing scientific efforts to discover a therapy or cure for this debilitating illness.

Treatment Options

The two primary types of these therapies are Pharmacological and Non-pharmacological methods.

Pharmaceutical Interventions:

Cholinesterase Inhibitors: These medications aid in raising acetylcholine levels, which are reduced in Alzheimer's patients. Cholinesterase inhibitors such as galantamine (Razadyne), rivastigmine (Exelon) and donepezil (Aricept) are often recommended.

Memantine, often known as Namenda, is an example of an NMDA Receptor Antagonist. It functions by controlling glutamate, an additional neurotransmitter connected to memory and learning. When Alzheimer's disease is mild to severe, memantine is often administered.

Non-Medicinal Interventions:

Cognitive Stimulation: Engaging in activities that enhance memory, reasoning and problem-solving abilities may help preserve cognitive function and delay the onset of cognitive decline. This covers social interactions, memory games and puzzles.

Exercise: Studies have shown that regular exercise enhances both general health and cognitive performance. Tai chi, swimming and walking are examples of exercises.

Healthy Diet: All aspects of health, including mental health, benefit from a balanced diet high in fruits, vegetables, whole grains, lean meats and healthy fats. Diets rich in antioxidants and omega-3 fatty acids, such as the Mediterranean diet, may help lower the risk of cognitive decline, according to some research.

Social Engagement: People with Alzheimer's disease may enhance their quality of life and protect their cognitive function by remaining socially engaged and maintaining their ties with friends and family.

Support for Carers: People with Alzheimer's disease greatly benefit from the assistance of carers. Carers may manage stress and better care for their loved ones by participating in support groups, getting respite care and learning about the condition.

People with Alzheimer's disease and their families collaborate closely with medical specialists to create a thorough treatment plan that takes into account their unique requirements and circumstances. In addition, scientists are always looking for novel therapies and interventions that might help people with Alzheimer's disease.

MEDICATIONS

Non-pharmacological Interventions

The goal of non-pharmacological therapies for Alzheimer's disease is to enhance the lives of those who are impacted by the illness. Alzheimer's has no known cure, although some treatments may help control symptoms and delay the illness's course.

The following are a few often used non-pharmacological interventions:

Activities like word games, puzzles, memory exercises and reminiscence therapy are examples of cognitive stimulation. Engaging in these activities may help prevent cognitive decline and preserve cognitive function.

Exercise: Research has shown that regular exercise may help people with Alzheimer's disease in many ways, including better mood, better sleep and an overall sense of well-being. In addition to slowing down cognitive ageing, exercise may lower the chance of acquiring other health problems including cardiovascular disease.

Nutritional Therapy: A well-balanced diet high in whole grains, fruits, vegetables, lean meats and healthy fats may help maintain general health and brain function. Antioxidants and omega-3 fatty acids are two examples of dietary supplements that may be helpful.

Social Engagement: Keeping up social relationships and taking part in social events might improve cognitive performance and lessen emotions of loneliness and despair. Alzheimer's patients and their carers might benefit from emotional support and useful guidance from support groups.

Music Therapy: For those suffering from Alzheimer's disease, listening to music or engaging in musical activities may bring back memories, lower anxiety and elevate mood. Additionally, music therapy may improve communication and encourage calm.

Art Therapy: Painting, sketching or creating are examples of creative hobbies that may provide people with Alzheimer's a feeling of achievement and a way to express themselves. A type of communication that may be used when verbal skills fail is art therapy.

Sensory Stimulation: Using techniques like aromatherapy, massage, or tactile stimulation to stimulate the senses may help people relax, become less agitated and feel better overall.

Environmental Changes: Providing a secure and encouraging atmosphere might assist people with Alzheimer's disease preserve their independence and lessen confusion. Decluttering living areas, putting up visual clues and reducing noise and distractions are a few examples of how to do this.

Pet Therapy: For those suffering from Alzheimer's disease, spending time with animals such as therapy dogs or cats, can be consoling and uplifting. It has been shown that pet therapy lowers agitation and raises mood.

Behavioural Interventions: Methods like redirection, validation therapy and behaviour modification strategies may help control difficult-to-control behaviours linked to Alzheimer's disease, such agitation, anger and wandering.

In cooperation with carers and healthcare providers, these non-pharmacological treatments have to be customised to the patient's requirements and preferences and used as a part of an all-encompassing care plan.

Alternative Therapies

A number of lifestyle modifications and complementary treatments have been investigated to help control symptoms and maybe halt the development of Alzheimer's disease. It's essential to remember that these strategies have to be included into thorough treatment plans and should always be reviewed with medical professionals.

Some researched Alternative therapies:

Dietary Adjustments: According to some studies, certain diets, such the MIND diet (which incorporates elements of the DASH diet with the Mediterranean diet), may help lower the risk of Alzheimer's disease or halt its development. These diets exclude red meat, processed meals and sweets while emphasising whole grains, fruits, vegetables, nuts, fish and olive oil.

Exercise: Studies have shown that engaging in regular physical exercise may improve brain health in a number of ways, including by lowering the risk of cognitive decline and perhaps delaying the onset of Alzheimer's disease. Strength training and cardiovascular activity, such cycling, swimming or walking, may both be beneficial.

Mental Stimulation: Those with Alzheimer's disease may have better quality of life and cognitive function if they participate in intellectually stimulating activities like reading, doing puzzles, picking up new skills or interacting with others.

Utilising Music to treat social, emotional or cognitive problems is known as music therapy. It has been shown to elevate mood, lessen agitation and anxiety and improve communication in Alzheimer's patients.

Art Therapy: Painting, sketching or sculpting are examples of creative exercises used in art therapy to help patients express their feelings and enhance their wellbeing.

It may be very helpful for those with Alzheimer's disease as a way to express themselves and communicate.

Acupuncture: According to some research, acupuncture may aid Alzheimer's patients' cognitive performance and lessen their behavioural symptoms. Nonetheless, further investigation is required to validate its efficacy.

Herbal Supplements: Studies have been conducted on the possible advantages of some herbal supplements, such as ginkgo biloba for Alzheimer's disease. The data is conflicting, thus these supplements should be taken cautiously since they may interfere with other prescriptions.

Mindfulness and Relaxation Techniques: Activities like yoga, tai chi, mindfulness meditation and deep breathing techniques may help lower stress, elevate mood and improve general wellbeing in both Alzheimer's patients and their carers.

Massage Treatment: For those suffering from Alzheimer's disease, massage treatment may assist lower agitation and elevate mood. Comfort and relaxation may be enhanced by gentle touch and massage.

Aromatherapy: According to some studies, using certain scents, such lavender or lemon balm, may help people with Alzheimer's disease sleep better and be less agitated.

Approach alternative treatments cautiously and seek medical advice before beginning any new therapy or intervention, even if they may help some people with Alzheimer's disease manage their symptoms and live better.

Caregiving Strategies

Although providing care for someone with Alzheimer's may be difficult, there are methods that can help both the Alzheimer's patient and the carer live better lives.

Here are some methods for providing care:

Become Informed: Get as much knowledge as you can on Alzheimer's illness. You can provide better care if you are aware of the disease's signs, progression and difficulties.

Create Routines: Alzheimer's patients often respond better to routines that have been created. Make an effort to maintain regular daily schedules for food, activities and sleep.

Establish a Safe Environment: Get rid of any potentially dangerous items or surfaces from the house, such sharp objects and slick flooring. Install grab bars and railings in the lavatory and any other places that may need them.

Promote Independence: Permit the Alzheimer's patient to take care of themselves as much as feasible. Give clear directions and divide work into small, doable segments.

Communicate Clearly: Use short phrases and basic language while speaking slowly and clearly. Keep your eyes open and wait for the Alzheimer's patient to speak.

Remember that Alzheimer's may alter behaviour and mood, so exercise patience and flexibility. Even under trying circumstances, strive to maintain your composure and exercise patience and flexibility.

Assist the Person with Alzheimer's Disease in Remembering Important Tasks and Appointments: Utilise memory aids like calendars, to-do lists and reminder notes.

Remain Active: Promote both mental and physical exercise. Walking, gardening, doing puzzles and listening to music are a few activities that might enhance mood and cognitive performance.

Take Care of Yourself: Providing care may be draining both mentally and physically. Take pauses, eat healthily, exercise often and ask friends, family or a support group for help when needed.

Seek Assistance: When you want assistance, don't be afraid to ask for it. Seek assistance from friends, family or neighbourhood resources. Think about becoming a member of a support group for Alzheimer's carers.

CREATING A SUPPORTIVE ENVIRONMENT

Communication Techniques

One way to create a friendly atmosphere for people with Alzheimer's disease is to use language that works.

Here are some tactics to think about:

Employ Simple Language: Make sure your words are precise and succinct. To get your point across, use short phrases and basic language.

Talk Clearly and Slowly: Don't talk too quickly. To make yourself more understandable to the person, talk more slowly and with clarity.

Maintain Eye Contact: Making eye contact with someone might aid in keeping them focused and attentive throughout a conversation. It also fosters trust and demonstrates respect.

Employ Nonverbal signals: To improve communication and transmit feelings or instructions, use nonverbal signals including body language, gestures and facial expressions.

Remain calm and patient: People with Alzheimer's disease may need more time to comprehend or react to stimuli. To prevent being frustrated or irritated during encounters, practise patience and maintain your composure.

Reduce Distractions: To assist the person in focusing on the discussion or work at hand, reduce background noise and other distractions.

Ask Basic Questions: To make it easy for the person to react, ask basic yes/no questions or provide options rather than complicated or open-ended inquiries.

Validate sentiments: Even if you don't really comprehend someone's point of view, you should nonetheless acknowledge and validate their sentiments. This promotes empathy and a feeling of community.

Use Visual Aids: To enhance spoken communication and promote comprehension, use visual aids like diagrams, photos or written directions.

Be Adaptable: Be ready to modify your communication approach in response to the requirements and reactions of the other person. Being adaptable is essential while communicating with Alzheimer's sufferers.

Repetition may be beneficial for memory retention. Repeat and reinforce this idea. As necessary, repeat important instructions or information and emphasise critical aspects all throughout the session.

Remain Positive: Throughout conversations, have a cheerful and encouraging demeanour. Encouragement and positive reinforcement may assist increase a person's confidence and level of participation.

Focus on sentiments, Not Facts: To maintain a good rapport, pay attention to validating the other person's sentiments and emotions rather than addressing factual mistakes or contradictions.

Use Familiar themes: Talking about or doing activities centred on the person's hobbies or familiar themes might assist to promote memory recall and engagement.

Seek Professional Assistance: For further help and resources, think about seeing a healthcare professional or specialist versed in Alzheimer's care if communication difficulties continue or become worse.

Try to provide a supportive atmosphere that improves the quality of life for people with Alzheimer's disease and promotes meaningful relationships and interactions by putting these communication skills into practice.

Managing Daily Activities

Changing habits and surroundings to accommodate a person with Alzheimer's disease entails managing their everyday activities. *Some tactics are:*

Create Routines: Adhere to regular daily plans for eating, taking medications and engaging in activities. Establishing routines lessens anxiety and confusion.

Divide Jobs into Easy Stages: Rather than giving someone a tonne of complicated instructions at once, divide a task into smaller, more manageable parts. As required, provide mild reminders and direction.

Give Visual Cues: To assist the individual in navigating their surroundings and remembering tasks, use visual aids like labels, signs or photos.

Promote Independence by letting the individual take care of oneself as much as possible, even if it takes longer or isn't done precisely. Assist and support them when required, but refrain from taking care of everything for them.

Establish a Secure Atmosphere: To avoid mishaps, clear the house of dangers and clutter. Grab bars, railings and other safety elements should be installed.

Simplify the Options: To prevent overwhelming the person, don't give them too many. Present straightforward choices and offer assistance when needed.

Provide Prompts and Reminders: Remind the individual about key chores or appointments by using timers, alarms or verbal signals.

Encourage Physical Activity: Frequent exercise helps lessen tension, elevate mood and enhance sleep quality. Select interesting and safe activities for the individual.

Serve Wholesome Meals: To promote general health and wellbeing, serve well-balanced meals and snacks all day long. Take food choices and any swallowing issues into account.

Organise and Distribute drugs according to a method to guarantee that they are taken accurately and on schedule. Take into account using automatic medicine dispensers or pill organisers.

Remain Connected by promoting social contact and involvement with loved ones. Continue to have deep conversations over the phone, in person or via video chat.

Observe Self-care: Prioritise your own physical and mental health since caring for someone with Alzheimer's may be taxing. When necessary, think about respite care and ask friends, family or support groups for assistance.

Legal and Financial Planning

For people with Alzheimer's disease and their families, financial and legal preparation is essential. *Here are some crucial things to remember:*

Establishing a power of attorney (POA) enables a chosen person—typically a family member or close friend, to handle financial and legal decisions on behalf of the person with Alzheimer's when they are unable to do so for themselves.

Advance Directives: These are legal papers that specify a person's preferences for medical care and last arrangements. Preferences for organ donation and life-sustaining procedures may fall under this category.

Will & Estate Planning: To guarantee that assets are allocated in accordance with the individual's desires, it's important to have a legitimate will in place. Determining beneficiaries and establishing trusts are other aspects of estate planning.

Financial Management: Keeping track of money might become harder as Alzheimer's gets worse. Limit access to big amounts of money, streamline accounts and set up recurring bill payments.

Planning for Long-Term Care: Alzheimer's often requires long-term care, which may be costly. To assist with these expenses, look into possibilities like Medicaid, long-term care insurance and veteran's benefits.

Guardianship/Conservatorship: If an Alzheimer's patient has not granted a power of attorney and is no longer able to make choices for themselves, the court may need to appoint a guardian or conservator to manage their finances and legal affairs.

Legal Assistance: To make sure that all relevant paperwork is in order and that legal concerns are handled correctly, speak with an attorney who specialises in elder law or estate planning.

Programmes for Financial Assistance: Research community and governmental initiatives that could provide support services or funds to people with Alzheimer's disease and their carers.

Examine and Update Frequently: To reflect any changes in circumstances or preferences, it's essential to examine and update legal and financial papers on a regular basis.

Support Services: To assist you through the difficulties of taking care of a loved one with Alzheimer's while handling legal and financial concerns, don't be afraid to look out for support services, such as carer support groups and respite care programmes.

It may be difficult to navigate the legal and financial planning aspects of Alzheimer's disease, but being proactive can reduce stress, guarantee that the person's desires are honoured and ensure that their financial affairs are properly handled.

Long-Term Care Options: Support Resources

Providing both practical and emotional support to a loved one suffering from Alzheimer's disease or another kind of dementia may be difficult. To make sure your loved one gets the finest care possible, it's important to investigate long-term care alternatives and available services.

Some alternatives to think about are:

In-home Care Services: A lot of families want to spend as much time as possible caring for a loved one who has Alzheimer's at home. In-home care services may help with companionship, medication management, everyday life tasks and more. These services may be customised to meet the requirements of your loved one and provide family carers with a break.

Memory Care Facilities: Individuals with Alzheimer's disease and other types of dementia are the focus of memory care facilities. These establishments provide a safe haven with dementia-aware personnel, planned activities to keep residents occupied and support services catered to the special needs of those suffering from memory loss.

Assisted life Facilities: For seniors who need assistance with everyday life tasks but do not require specialised nursing care, assisted living facilities provide lodging, food, personal care assistance and support services. Specialised memory care units are available in some assisted living homes for those suffering from dementia and Alzheimer's.

Nursing Homes: For those who need more help with daily living tasks and medical care, nursing homes provide competent nursing care around-the-clock. Specialised dementia care programmes or memory care facilities are available in some nursing homes.

Adult Day Programmes: During the day, adults with dementia or Alzheimer's disease may participate in scheduled activities, socialisation and supervision. These programmes may provide family carers a break and give dementia patients chances for interaction and stimulation.

Support Groups: Support groups provide a feeling of community, practical guidance and emotional support to carers of people with Alzheimer's disease. These groups may take place in person or virtually and they can be led by medical experts, charitable organisations or community centres.

Respite Care: Respite care services provide people with Alzheimer's disease short-term, in-home care, relieving family carers of some of their caregiving duties. Residential care institutions, adult day programmes and in-home care organisations may all make arrangements for this.

Telemedicine and Internet Resources: For people with Alzheimer's disease, telemedicine services may provide remote medical treatment and consultations, particularly for medication management and health monitoring. For carers and those who have Alzheimer's, there are also a plethora of internet resources, instructional materials and support forums at their disposal.

Evaluate each loved one's unique requirements, preferences and financial situation when thinking about long-term care alternatives for a person with Alzheimer's.

You may make educated choices about the optimal care plan for your loved one by navigating the various alternatives with the assistance of social workers, elder care experts and healthcare professionals.

SHORT PERIOD CARE SERVICES

Online Resources and Helplines

It's essential to support people with Alzheimer's disease and those who care for them; there are a number of online sites and hotlines that may provide support, information and aid. These reliable sources are listed below:

The Alzheimer's Association

Online at **alz.org**
1-800-272-3900 is the helpline.
offers a multitude of resources, teaching materials, support groups, tools for carers and research updates for people with Alzheimer's disease.

The American Foundation on Alzheimer's (AFA):

https://alzfdn.org
Contact number: **1-866-232-8484**

provides care consultations, educational materials and
support services for people with Alzheimer's disease and
their family.

NIA, the National Institute on Ageing:

Nia.nih.gov/alzheimers is the website.
offers thorough details about Alzheimer's disease,
including updates on research and information on
diagnosis, caring and therapy.

Alliance of Family Carers:

URL: caregiver.org
provides a number of tools and services, such as caring
advice, instructional materials and online forums, for
family carers.

Alzheimers.net:

https://alzheimers.net

offers community resources, advice for carers, solutions
for memory care and information about Alzheimer's
disease.

The CAN (Carers Action Network):

URL: caregiveraction.org
provides tools and assistance for family carers, including
advocacy campaigns, instructional materials and online
support groups.

Memory Maintenance:

MemoryCare.org is the website.
offers specialist memory care services, such as educational
programmes, carer support and diagnostic assessments.

Central Dementia Care:

dementiacarecentral.com is the website.

provides information about Alzheimer's and dementia, including financial and legal preparation, caring techniques and residential care choices.

These may provide Alzheimer's patients and their carers with important support, knowledge and direction. Healthcare providers and neighbourhood organisations may also be able to give further support and assistance based on individual requirements.

Lifestyle Considerations

Lifestyle factors are crucial for individuals with Alzheimer's disease to manage symptoms, maintain quality of life and **potentially slow** the progression of the disease.

A healthy diet rich in fruits, vegetables, whole grains, lean proteins and healthy fats can support overall health and reduce the risk of chronic conditions associated with Alzheimer's disease.

Regular exercise, such as aerobic, strength training and flexibility exercises, can improve mood, reduce stress and promote overall well-being. Mental stimulation, such as puzzles, games, reading and hobbies, can help maintain cognitive function and delay cognitive decline.

Social engagement can reduce feelings of isolation and improve mood. Regular sleep, with good sleep hygiene, can improve sleep quality and cognitive function. Stress management, such as deep breathing exercises, meditation, yoga or listening to music, can negatively impact cognitive function and overall well-being.

Establishing a daily routine and structure can reduce confusion and agitation. Safety precautions, such as installing handrails and using assistive devices, are essential to prevent accidents and injuries.

Effective medication management requires collaboration with healthcare professionals and a strong support system for both the individual and their caregivers is important.

Tailoring lifestyle interventions to the individual's preferences, abilities and stage of Alzheimer's disease is essential.

Consulting with healthcare professionals can help develop a comprehensive care plan that addresses the unique needs of each person with Alzheimer's disease.

DIET AND NUTRITION

Maintaining a balanced diet and enough nutrition is mandatory for Alzheimer's sufferers in order to support their general health and maybe reduce the disease's development.

These dietary guidelines are can be really helpful:

The Mediterranean Diet is high in whole grains, nuts, seeds, fruits, vegetables and heart-healthy fats like olive oil. It also entails limiting red meat and sweets and consuming fish and poultry in moderation. Alzheimer's disease and cognitive impairment have been linked to a decreased risk of Alzheimer's diet.

Omega-3 Fatty Acids: Consuming foods high in omega-3 fatty acids, such walnuts, flaxseeds, chia seeds and fatty fish (salmon, mackerel and sardines), may help maintain brain function and lower inflammation.

Foods High in Antioxidants: Antioxidants aid in defending cells against harm from free radicals. Berries (strawberries, raspberries and blueberries), dark leafy greens (kale, spinach) and vibrant veggies (carrots, bell peppers and tomatoes) are foods rich in antioxidants.

Vitamin E: Research indicates that vitamin E may be able to slow down Alzheimer's disease's course. Avocados, spinach, sunflower seeds, almonds and sunflower seeds are good sources of vitamin E.

Vitamins B: B vitamins, especially B6, B12 and folate, are important for maintaining brain function and may also lower homocysteine levels, which are connected to cognitive decline. Fish, poultry, eggs, dairy products, leafy greens and fortified cereals are foods high in B vitamins.

Restrict Sugary Foods and Processed Carbohydrates: Diets high in sugar and refined carbs may aggravate insulin resistance and inflammation, both of which are harmful to the health of the brain. Limit your intake of processed snacks, drinks and sugary meals.

Hydration: Sufficient hydration is critical for both general health and mental performance. Promote drinking water and other liquids on a regular basis throughout the day.

Small, Regular Meals: Eating big meals or remembering to eat might be challenging for some Alzheimer's patients. In order to provide sufficient nutrition throughout the day, smaller, more frequent meals and snacks should be provided.

Think About Texture Modifications: People may have difficulties swallowing or chewing as their Alzheimer's condition worsens. When necessary, adjust the texture of food by pureeing it or presenting it in a soft, approachable form.

Speak with a Registered Dietitian: Depending on their age, gender, weight and general health, each person may have different dietary requirements. Alzheimer's patients and their carers may get customised advice and assistance from a trained nutritionist.

Understand that while maintaining a balanced diet might enhance general wellbeing, it cannot treat Alzheimer's disease.

PHYSICAL EXERCISE

Physical Exercise best for Alzheimer's patients

The benefits of physical activity for those with Alzheimer's disease are enormous. Enhancing mood, lowering anxiety and despair, improving cognitive function and possibly delaying the course of the illness are all possible benefits. But it's important to choose activities that are secure and suitable for the person's skills and Alzheimer's stage.

The following activities are usually seen to be beneficial:

Walking: Easily customised to an individual's ability, walking is a straightforward, low-impact workout. It strengthens muscles, enhances cardiovascular health and aids in maintaining mobility.

Swimming: Since swimming is easy on the joints and gives your whole body a workout, it's an excellent alternative for those with Alzheimer's. It may enhance coordination, physical strength and cardiovascular health.

Tai Chi: Tai Chi is a kind of mind-body training that focuses on deep breathing and fluid, leisurely motions. It has been shown to enhance elderly persons' balance, flexibility and cognitive performance, including Alzheimer's patients.

Yoga: Yoga promotes general health and well-being by combining physical postures, breathing techniques, and meditation. Strength, balance, flexibility and mood may all be enhanced by it.

Chair Exercises: These might be a terrific alternative for those who are unable to stand for extended periods of time or who have restricted mobility. These workouts are done while sitting on a chair and include light movements and stretches.

Dancing: Dancing is an enjoyable kind of exercise that improves mood, balance and coordination. Dancing may be customised to suit the skills and tastes of the person; it can be ballroom, line or just dancing to music at home.

Before beginning any fitness programme, it's essential to speak with a healthcare provider, particularly for those who have Alzheimer's disease.

Based on the person's ability, medical history, also illness stage - they may assist in determining the best workouts.

Carers should also guarantee the safety and efficacy of the exercise regimen by offering monitoring and assistance as required.

MENTAL STIMULATION

For Alzheimer's patients, mental stimulation is mandatory for maintaining cognitive function and quality of life.

Here are some activities and techniques that might help:

Games & Puzzles: Playing board games, jigsaw puzzles, crosswords and Sudoku may assist sharpen cognitive abilities and engage the mind.

Memory Exercises: Easy memory exercises that aid with short-term memory include identifying items in a room, remembering prior experiences, and playing memory games.

Music: Playing an instrument or listening to well-known music may trigger memories and feelings, stimulating the mind and elevating mood. This is known as music therapy.

Art & Creativity: Painting, sketching or creating are examples of creative hobbies that might help Alzheimer's sufferers feel accomplished and stimulate their minds.

Storytelling and Reading: Giving Alzheimer's sufferers the opportunity to read or read aloud to them may assist, engage and excite their minds.

Exercise: Research has shown that regular exercise enhances cognitive function and slows the development of Alzheimer's disease. Exercises like yoga, swimming and walking might be helpful.

Social Interaction: Socialising with friends, relatives or engaging in group activities may give mental stimulation and emotional support for Alzheimer's sufferers.

Learning New Skills: Introducing Alzheimer's patients to new hobbies or skills, like cooking, gardening or learning to play an instrument, can help increase their sense of self-worth and brain stimulation.

Reminiscence Therapy: Using images, films or narratives to relive old events may assist jog memory and provide a feeling of continuity and identity.

Technology-Based Activities: Alzheimer's sufferers may benefit from mental stimulation by using tablets or PCs to play brain-training games, video chat with loved ones or access educational materials.

Activities should be customised to the person's interests, capabilities, and disease stage. A supportive and motivating atmosphere should also be provided.

Also, caregivers should be patient and empathetic, offering aid and encouragement as required.

COPING WITH CHALLENGES

Dealing with Behavioural Symptoms

Providing care for individuals with Alzheimer's disease may be difficult, particularly when behavioural signs are present.

The following tactics may be used to assist control these behaviours:

Maintain a Routine: Having a regular daily schedule may assist to provide structure and predictability to life, which can help to lessen confusion and anxiety.

Reduce clutter, noise and distractions to create a peaceful atmosphere. Employ calming hues and gentle lighting to provide a tranquil environment.

Promote Exercise: Frequent exercise helps elevate mood and lessen tension. Exercises in a chair, walking and mild stretching may all be helpful.

Offer Meaningful Activities: Involve the patient in pursuits that align with their passions and skills, such crossword puzzles, arts and crafts, gardening or music listening. Engaging in these hobbies may provide both excitement and a feeling of achievement.

Employ Distraction Techniques: Offer an alternative activity or discussion subject to divert the patient's focus from upsetting behaviours.

Practice Validation: Give the person's experiences and emotions your acknowledgement, even if they don't make sense or appear out of touch with reality. Refrain from disputing or refuting their opinions.

See to Safety: To ensure safety, get rid of any potentially dangerous items or trip hazards from the area. If roaming is an issue, think about installing locks or alarms on doors and windows.

Keep an eye on your Medications: mSome drugs may interfere with other drugs or exacerbate behavioural issues. Review the patient's medication schedule on a frequent basis in close collaboration with their healthcare practitioner.

Comfort and Reassurance: In times of bewilderment or anxiety, provide the patient with comfort and reassurance. A feeling of security may be aided by familiar things, comforting words and gentle touch.

Embrace Support: It may be emotionally and physically exhausting to care for someone who has Alzheimer's. To help you deal with the difficulties, don't be afraid to ask friends, family, support groups or professional carers for assistance.

Think About Getting Professional Help: Speak with a medical expert who specialises in Alzheimer's treatment if behavioural symptoms worsen or become difficult to control. They may provide direction, help with medicine administration, and extra resources to help the patient and the carer.

Do Note that each person with Alzheimer's disease is different, so what works for one may not work for another. In order to care for someone with Alzheimer's and manage their behavioural symptoms, it is essential to have patience, flexibility and empathy.

Addressing Caregiver Stress

For carers, taking care of a loved one with Alzheimer's disease may be emotionally and physically draining. These techniques may be used to reduce carer stress:

Become Informed: Carers can foresee difficulties and create coping mechanisms by having a thorough understanding of the course of Alzheimer's disease. A portion of the anxiety and uncertainty might be reduced by knowing what to anticipate.

Seek Help: You may feel validated and part of a community by joining a support group for carers of Alzheimer's patients. It may be very reassuring to share stories and guidance with those who are experiencing comparable circumstances.

Take Breaks: Self-care should be a top priority for carers. It's important to take frequent pauses to refuel, rest and partake in enjoyable and soothing activities. To offer respite care, enlist the assistance of friends, family or hired carers.

Have Reasonable Expectations: Acknowledge that you have no power over or ability to stop Alzheimer's from becoming worse. Be kind to yourself when things don't work out the way you had hoped and set reasonable expectations for both you and your loved one.

Use Stress-Reduction Strategies: Include stress-relieving activities in your everyday routine, such as yoga, meditation, deep breathing or mindfulness. These techniques may aid in calming down and reducing anxiety.

Maintain a Healthy Lifestyle: Make sleep a priority, eat a balanced diet and get frequent exercise. Maintaining your physical well-being may increase your ability to withstand stress and assist you in managing the difficulties of providing care.

Effective Communication: Maintain lines of communication open with family, friends and other support systems as well as healthcare professionals. Communicate honestly about your wants, worries and

limits. When you need assistance, don't be afraid to ask for
it.

Celebrate Little Victories: With your loved one,
acknowledge and rejoice in little victories and happy
moments, no matter how brief they may be. Discovering
happy moments may provide a counterpoint to the
challenges of providing care.

Think About Professional Assistance: If providing care
becomes too much or unmanageable, think about
contacting a professional. A portion of the load on family
carers may be reduced by using assisted living
communities, adult day care centres or in-home carers.

Future Care Requirements: Project future care
requirements and develop strategies in line with them.
This might include talking with your loved one and other
family members about your end-of-life desires as well as
making financial and legal plans.

Do prioritise your well-being when caring for a loved one with Alzheimer's disease and keep in mind that carer stress is common.

Carers may better manage stress and offer their loved ones high-quality care by putting these methods into practice and getting help when they need it.

Planning for Transitions in Care

Providing care for an individual with Alzheimer's disease necessitates organising different care transitions as the illness advances.

Some crucial things for carers to think about:

Early Planning: As the condition progresses, it is essential to begin preparing for care transitions as soon as possible. This gives time for option research, decision-making and making sure the Alzheimer's patient participates in the process as much as possible while they are still able to do so.

Health Care Proxy and Advance Directives: While
the Alzheimer's patient is still able to make thoughtful
choices, assist them in appointing a healthcare proxy and
drafting advance directives. These agreements outline
their choices for healthcare and name a proxy for them in
the event that they are unable to make decisions for
themselves.

Comprehending the Illness Progression: Because
Alzheimer's disease progresses over time, a person's care
requirements will also vary. It is important for carers to
become knowledgeable about the many phases of
Alzheimer's disease and the symptoms and difficulties that
come with each stage.

Support Services: To assist manage caregiving
obligations and deal with the emotional and physical
strains of caring for someone with Alzheimer's, make use
of support services including Alzheimer's organisations,
support groups and respite care.

In-Home Care: With the assistance of family members or in-home carers, an individual with Alzheimer's disease may be able to live at home in the early stages of the disease. More care may be required when the illness worsens in order to protect the patient's health and safety.

Memory Care Facilities: When a person's care demands go beyond what can be safely and successfully given at home, think about moving them into a memory care facility that specialises in Alzheimer's and dementia care. Specialised services and a comforting atmosphere catered to the particular requirements of people with Alzheimer's disease are provided by memory care facilities.

Legal and Financial Planning: As an individual's cognitive skills deteriorate, work with a legal or financial counsellor to set up guardianship, power of attorney, and other legal arrangements to handle their affairs.

Frequent Evaluations: Arrange for regular evaluations with medical specialists to track the patient's status and modify the treatment plan as necessary. Therapy, medication management and other treatments aimed at treating symptoms and enhancing quality of life may be part of this.

End-of-Life Planning: Discuss last wants and preferences, such as those pertaining to hospice care, life-sustaining medical treatments and funeral plans. Make sure to include these choices in advance directives and let family members and medical professionals know about them.

Self-Care: In order to prevent burnout and offer their loved one with Alzheimer's the best care possible, carers must put their own physical and emotional well-being first. This might include asking for help from friends, family and medical experts, taking breaks, also requesting respite care.

Carers may more effectively handle the difficulties of caring for a person with Alzheimer's disease and guarantee the patient gets the best care possible throughout the illness's course by proactively planning for care transitions and gaining access to the right support resources.

RESEARCH AND FUTURE DIRECTIONS

Current Research Trends

There has been a great deal of and continuous study conducted on Alzheimer's disease (AD), with a focus on many different facets of the illness, such as its pathology, risk factors, early identification, therapy and prevention.

Here are a few recent developments in the subject of research:

Amyloid Beta and Tau Proteins: Two of the main characteristics of Alzheimer's disease are tangles of tau proteins and amyloid beta plaques. Their function in the pathophysiological process and possible treatment targets targeted at preventing their build-up or encouraging their clearance are still being studied.

Genetics and Risk Factors: Research on genetics has linked a number of genes, notably the APOE gene, to a higher chance of Alzheimer's disease. Scientists are examining the potential interactions between these genetic markers and other risk factors, including age, lifestyle and environmental factors.

Early Detection and Diagnosis: Finding ways to identify Alzheimer's disease and make the diagnosis before symptoms appear is becoming more and more important.

This involves identifying those who are at risk or in the early stages of the illness via the use of biomarkers such as imaging methods (such as PET scans) and blood-based biomarkers.

Precision Medicine Approaches: Personalised or precision medicine approaches to Alzheimer's disease are becoming more and more popular due to advances in biomarker research and genetics. Therapeutic approaches may be improved by customising care based on a patient's genetic profile, biomarker status and other variables.

Vaccines and Immunotherapy: Immunotherapy techniques, such as the creation of antibodies that target the tau or amyloid beta proteins, are being investigated as possible Alzheimer's disease therapies. Researchers are also looking at the possibility of vaccines to stop or delay the disease's course.

Lifestyle Interventions: A number of lifestyle variables have been linked to an increased risk of Alzheimer's disease, including nutrition, exercise, social interaction and cognitive stimulation. In order to create therapies that might lower the risk of cognitive decline or postpone its commencement, research is being done to better understand how these variables affect brain health.

Drug discovery and Clinical Trials: Research into novel pharmacological therapies for Alzheimer's disease is ongoing, with a focus on small molecule medications that target several facets of the disease's pathology. Trials in humans are being conducted to assess the effectiveness and safety of these possible remedies.

Non-pharmacological Interventions: In addition to medication therapies, non-pharmacological interventions are being researched for their potential to enhance cognitive function and quality of life in Alzheimer's disease patients. These interventions include cognitive training, physical exercise regimens and lifestyle changes.

Digital Health Technologies: Wearables, smartphone applications and remote monitoring systems are just a few examples of the digital health technologies that are becoming more and more popular in Alzheimer's research. These technologies have the potential to improve early diagnosis, track the course of illness and provide more individualised and easily available therapies.

Multimodal Approaches: Due to the intricacy of Alzheimer's disease, scientists are looking more closely at multimodal strategies that concurrently address many disease pathological elements. Combining several therapy or treatment methods may have a positive synergistic impact and improve patient results.

There are constant attempts to better understand the illness's causes, find new therapeutic targets and create efficient preventative and therapy measures in the dynamic and diverse area of Alzheimer's disease research.

It will need cooperation between scientists, physicians, business partners and advocacy organisations to further our understanding and eventually discover a treatment for Alzheimer's disease.

Clinical Trials

Numerous clinical studies have been conducted on Alzheimer's disease, a neurodegenerative condition, with the goal of understanding its underlying causes, creating efficient therapies and investigating possible preventative measures. Alzheimer's disease clinical trials often fall into many categories:

Drug trials: These studies examine the effectiveness of novel or already available pharmaceuticals in treating the symptoms of Alzheimer's disease, delaying the advancement of the illness or addressing underlying pathology such as the buildup of tau or beta-amyloid proteins.

Trials for Prevention: These studies focus on people who are not yet suffering from Alzheimer's disease but who are at risk due to a genetic susceptibility or a family history. Finding treatments that could postpone or stop the development of symptoms is the aim.

Behavioural Interventions: Studies may look at how well lifestyle interventions, such fitness regimens, mental training, food modifications and social interaction, might enhance cognitive function or impede the course of a disease.

Diagnostic Trials: The goal of these studies is to create
and validate biomarkers or imaging methods that may be
used to accurately diagnose Alzheimer's disease early on,
which is essential for prompt intervention and therapy.

Combination Therapy studies aim to target several
pathways involved in the disease process by combining
different medications or therapies. This approach is
chosen because of the complicated nature of Alzheimer's
disease.

Gene Therapy Trials: Targeting certain genetic mutations
linked to family types of Alzheimer's disease, gene therapy
techniques are being investigated in light of advancements
in genetic research.

Trials of Immunotherapy: These studies look at the use
of vaccines or antibodies to target and eliminate tau or
beta-amyloid protein clumps from the brain in an effort to
delay the course of illness.

Non-Pharmacological Trials: These studies assess non-pharmacological treatments, such as art therapy, music therapy, sensory stimulation and other complementary methods, to enhance quality of life and control behavioural symptoms in Alzheimer's disease patients.

NOTE that despite the fact that Alzheimer's disease has been the subject of several clinical studies, developing effective therapies has proved difficult and has resulted in multiple failures.

Ongoing research, however, raises hopes for new discoveries and deepens our knowledge of the illness.

Clinical trial registries, research institutes and healthcare providers are good places to start looking for options for anybody interested in taking part in Alzheimer's disease clinical studies.

CONCLUSION AND ADDITIONAL TIPS

Importance of Self-Care

For both those who are caring for someone with Alzheimer's disease and the person themselves, self-care is vital.

The following justifies the importance of self-care in the management of Alzheimer's disease:

Maintaining Physical Health: Three key components of self-care include eating a balanced diet, obtaining adequate sleep and participating in regular physical exercise. Exercise has been shown to enhance cognitive performance and lower the likelihood of deterioration in Alzheimer's patients.

Sleep and a healthy diet also contribute to general wellbeing and may aid with symptom management.

Emotional Well-Being: Both the person with the diagnosis and their carers may experience emotional strain as a result of Alzheimer's disease. Stress may be decreased and mood can be elevated by engaging in self-care practices including meditation, relaxation methods and hobby or interest pursuits.

In order to avoid burnout, carers must take breaks and look for outside help.

Cognitive Stimulation: Taking part in cognitively demanding activities may assist extend cognitive function and slow down the ageing process. This might include reading, solving riddles or picking up new abilities.

Also, carers may provide cognitive stimulation by conversing, reflecting or participating in activities with their care recipients.

Social Interaction: In order to preserve their quality of life, people with Alzheimer's disease must continue to be socially linked. Attending support groups, hanging out with friends and family and engaging in social activities may all help to lessen feelings of loneliness and provide emotional support.

To promote the well-being of the person, carers need to support and foster social contacts.

Structure and Routine: People with Alzheimer's disease may feel more stable and predictable if they are able to establish and stick to a daily schedule. This may enhance general functioning and lessen confusion and anxiety. In order to keep daily activities structured and routines intact, carers are important.

Safety and Hygiene: Taking care of oneself also includes taking care of fundamental requirements like grooming, safety, and personal hygiene. As their condition worsens, people with Alzheimer's may need help with these duties. In addition to ensuring the person's personal care requirements are satisfied, carers should make sure the environment is secure and encouraging.

Seeking Support: Getting help from medical experts, support groups and local resources is beneficial for both Alzheimer's patients and the people who care for them.

This may provide helpful advice, emotional support and important information all throughout the Alzheimer's disease journey.

So therefore, maintaining physical health, emotional stability, cognitive function, social ties and an overall quality of life for people with Alzheimer's disease and their carers depends on self-care.

People may improve their well-being and more effectively handle the difficulties brought on by Alzheimer's disease by making self-care activities a priority.

Hope and Resilience in the Journey

The slogan **"Alzheimer's Disease: Hope and Resilience in the Journey"** sums up the continuous fight against Alzheimer's disease, a neurodegenerative condition that mostly affects the elderly and progressively deteriorates memory and cognitive function.

There is hope and resiliency in the path of those impacted by Alzheimer's, as well as their loved ones and carers, despite the disease's terrible effects.

There is hope because of the continuous study and knowledge of the illness, as well as possible interventions and therapies that might stop the illness from progressing or at least slow it down. In an effort to enhance the quality of life for those suffering with Alzheimer's disease, a plethora of research is investigating a range of options, including lifestyle modifications and medication therapy.

When people and families deal with the difficulties brought on by Alzheimer's with fortitude, flexibility and resolve, they are exhibiting resilience. Even while caring for someone with Alzheimer's brings challenges, many carers manage the journey with dignity and compassion, asking for help from medical experts, support groups and local resources.

Furthermore, those who have Alzheimer's disease themselves frequently exhibit incredible bravery and tenacity in the face of cognitive deterioration, demonstrating resilience.

For as long as possible, they keep their relationships with their loved ones intact, appreciate their memories and find delight in the little things in life.

Resilience and hope go hand in hand on the Alzheimer's journey, supporting patients and their families through highs and lows, encouraging them to keep moving ahead and reassuring them that they are not fighting this difficult illness alone.

"Every moment that is lost while dealing with Alzheimer's disease is evidence of inner power.

We discover fortitude, bravery and the unflinching will to savour each moment as it comes along while accepting the road with grace and hope with every new difficulty."